I0450180

Herbal Antibiotics:

Natural Remedies and Herbal Recipes to Prevent, Treat and Heal Illnesses and Common Allergies

By

Debra Helton

ISBN-13: 978-1505615449

Table of Contents

Herbal Antibiotics: Natural Remedies and Herbal Recipes to Prevent, Treat and Heal Illnesses and Common Allergies

By Debra Helton

© Copyright 2014 Debra Helton

Reproduction or translation of any part of this work beyond that permitted by section 107 or 108 of the 1976 United States Copyright Act without permission of the copyright owner is unlawful. Requests for permission or further information should be addressed to the author.

This publication is designed to provide accurate and authoritative information in regard to the subject matter covered. This work is sold with the understanding that the publisher is not engaged in rendering legal, accounting, or other professional services. If legal advice or other expert assistance is required, the services of a competent professional person should be sought.

First Published, 2014

Printed in the United States of America

Introduction

If you have any concerns regarding the dangers of antibiotics, you might be someone that is interested to know a variety of antibiotic remedies available around the world you can use. Certain herbs as well as other potent antibiotic substances could relieve your signs fast and naturally. The best thing is that you can easily get those without a prescription. Learn the basics in regards of herbal natural antibiotics and get recipes described in this book to get started. Making such remedies generally is a fun and instructive solution to involve everyone in your house.

They are simply organic. You don't need to concern regarding odd chemical substances that come with many negative side effects. If you prepare such remedies in your own home, it is you that will be capable to control exactly all of them. It is possible for you to make use of completely natural mechanisms. You can make use of the essential oils you have a preference the fragrance and many more. Making natural cure costs becomes far lower than purchasing them. For anyone who is a fan of natural treatments, you may end up being just how simple and cheap they're to make in your own home. This guide will tell you about natural remedies and herbal recipes that can prevent and heal illnesses and common allergies.

Chapter 1. Allergies

There are numerous people that experiencing some form of allergy. In fact, it is usually a food allergy, or some sort of pet allergy. There could be an allergic reaction to pollen within the air. When it comes to a mild allergy, it might make along with a severe allergy that is usually life threatening. Luckily the good thing is, there are natural and organic and herbal remedies that help stop Hypersensitivity attacks and manage the symptoms.

To control allergy symptoms, you should come about the three things. Firstly, you should spot what you tend to be allergic to in order to avoid it whenever likely and make out what sort of defensive remedies to make use of. The next thing is, you utilize solutions to make the body's defense mechanism stronger to prevent problems. Finally, use them to lessen the severity associated with an allergy hit and cure it.

Allergy sufferers through the entire centuries have considered warm tea to supply help for a stuffy nose as well as irritated mucous walls, and one most useful for symptom alleviation is peppermint herbal tea. Its benefits prolong well ahead of its tasty odor. The oil acts like a decongestant. Elements in peppermint consist of anti-inflammatory and moderate antibacterial elements.

1. For making peppermint tea, get 1/2 Oz dried leaves of peppermint inside a 1-quart pot. Fill 2/3rd of the pot with hot water, and sheer for five minutes a few minutes. Take the steam for additional advantage. Let it cool, then strain, sweeten and consume.

You can make use of eucalyptus oil with regard to seasonal allergy cure in several ways. It is possible for you to put more than a few drops into the Neti Container, inhale it using a diffuser. You can also apply it in the laundry detergent. You should know that this antimicrobial agent. Mix eucalyptus essential oil. Now you need to rub it on the chest and at the rear of your ears in addition to diffuse it within the air throughout the day. Use it while you are sleeping.

2. Red clover, fennel, and Calendula preserve mucous hydrated to assist ward off Contamination. Nettle is an all natural, an organic and natural antihistamine. Peppermint and Spearmint help open airways. Lavender provides

antiseptic elements in the event that contamination creeps in. Eyebright is of great help for a whole Variety of sinus problems and especially beneficial to hay fever. Yerba Santa is an herbal item that acts being an expectorant, eliminating mucous in addition to phlegm.

When you're making herbal tea with regard to medicinal use, just be sure you get ready a powerful decoction. For just one 8-oz serving, employ two to three tablespoons of natural herbs. To generate a superior amount to swallow the whole day, then you need to make the tea within a big container.

3. Coconut oil allows you to ease rashes you skin offers. Put in a couple of drops of lemon and apply at regions.

4. Seeds of poppy are thought to be very effective in dealing with skin allergies. Get 1 table spoon of poppy seeds. Mix using a bit of water in order to create a paste. Include 1 tsp of such juice into it and apply towards the affected skin.

5. Castor oil is effective for food allergies. Eat 1 tsp of oil per day on a bare stomach. The oil really helps to calm the gastrointestinal tract by reducing discomfort.

6. Quercetin is considered to be among the finest natural remedies intended for allergies. This provides to be natural anti-histamine. It can prevent an allergic attack. Quercetin is seen in foods like parsley, apples, and onions. Olive oil, grapes and Dark berries, also include quercetin.

Chapter 2. Abdominal Pain

Chamomile plant comes with the element of suppressing and numbing the swollen gases and pain in the belly. The plant is as well identified to manipulate diarrhea, in particular in children. It's probably taken when anyone has a disturb abdomen. It's identified to have some oil that can absorb the infected gas in your belly. Chamomile can improve the leisure of the muscle tissues, hence dropping the jagged pangs.

Use chamomile as part of the treatment for a belly ache. It is boiled and the mixture is taken out from drinking as tea. Chamomile may be combined with honey or some other aromas to discourage the unpleasantness of the fluid.

Fennel

This herb is used to treat many ailments apart from the stomach agony. Fennel has been used for a lengthy period, especially with the aid of the Chinese. It's identified to have nutrition, potassium, folic acid, and fibers, which certainly aid in acid stomach. It is as well recognized to include the disturb stomach consequently of swelling. It can be used to ease flatulence via the rectum. Essentially the mightiest part of this plant is the seed. This is a beneficial home therapy for the difficulty.

Use fennel as a healing for abdominal discomfort. You can use it in both tea and food. Take 2 grams of fennel. It must be taken a minimum of two times a day. Take after each meal like a chewing gum. This helps in quicker absorption of the food.

Ginger

Essentially the most vigorous constituents of the ginger are the roots and the stem. It is famous to incorporate antacid property properties. It contains oil that is beneficial in decreasing the upset belly as good because the infection. It is recognized to incorporate some substances that may be very caring to pregnant females, because it can decrease the vomiting. The strong phenol located within the ginger roots can help relieve the metabolism through taking up the fuel derived within the digestion procedure.

The basis or stem will have to be washed fully and peeled off prior to boiling. You can boil it for 15 minutes to get the enzymes. To cut the bitterness, mix it with 2 teaspoons of honey. Consume the mixture after each meal unless the belly ache is over. It is considered one of the quality common therapies for a stomach problem. It must be delivered in meals as a weight loss plan for the belly pain.

Mint

This herb has been some of the outstanding home cures for belly pains. It's identified to contain homes that supporting the digestion. You can use it for your stomach pain. Some of the illnesses you can use the ginger are indigestion, vomiting, menstrual cramps and stomach aches. It can help soothe the belly from any infection that will occur after the absorption. It can also be very valuable for little children because it helps stomach pain.

Use mint as a cure for abdominal pain. The plant may also be taken in a raw form. Chew it after every meal. To use mint, you should boil it. Then, use the juice with tea. You must no longer use it with milk, because it has been recognized that milk makes it much less powerful. The concoction will have to now be taken at once, however, sipping for a couple of hours is suggested.

Yogurt

It contains a few beneficial bacteria that are extremely valuable for the body. There are many microorganisms that help break down the foods into little pieces so the body can absorb easily. The moment the acid is available for longer in your stomach, it causes a few harms to the abdominal partition, making your belly distress. These micro organisms as well help relieve the belly pain. Yogurt has the capability to catalyze the acid influx. It is also in use to weight loss programs.

Use yogurt as a cure for stomach soreness. Yogurt can also be taken a couple of minutes after consuming a meal. It's worthwhile to take yogurt most effective after consuming a meal that's identified to acquire to digest; accordingly it is compatible for serious diets.

Licorice

You can use it in the treatment of stomach soreness. It contains a number of properties that sustain to reduce the acid in the stomach and intestines. With the mucous, it can dilute the acid. In addition, it is also well known to absorb the seditious fuel created in your stomach. It can efficiently ease the pain the stomach brings.

Boil the plant for about sixteen minutes to take out the entire needed enzymes in the answer. Other objects such as honey can be brought to expand its efficiency and increase its taste. Use 250 ml after each meal. Take it at a minimum of two times a day, whatever the meals. When a typical belly pain comes, you can use it to relive the acidity within the stomach.

Chapter 2. Acidity

Almonds

Almonds are extremely wealthy in diet and different vitamins and minerals like calcium, iron, phosphorus, and magnesium. Using almonds can help cure your burning sensation occurred because of the acidity. It helps neutralize the acid. They are a just right source of ordinary medication of acidity. Eat 4-5 faded almonds after each and every meal to stop the happening of acidity.

Yogurt

It includes an excessive degree of potassium, calcium, vitamin B12 and B2 and magnesium. It helps enable digestion. For this reason, it eases acidity. Considering the fact that it allows absorption of proteins, hence using it no longer causes indigestion. To treat your acidity, you can also consume it. Take yogurt after each meal. With some sugar, get yoghurt when experiencing acidity.

Ginger

It comprises nutrition C, protein, iron, calcium, phosphorus, manganese, and folic acid. It is enormously helpful in bettering the working of the absorption procedure. It allows simplifying proteins and graceful absorption of fatty acids. If you are experiencing bloating, take ginger. It's truly considered one of the most excellent natural home remedies to cure acidity.

Coriander

Coriander is very effective in the treatment of a wide verity of diseases you can use at home. You can easily cure your several most common problems with it. The most common health problems it can relive are skin inflammation, mouth ulcers, diarrhea, high cholesterol, menstrual, anemia, and digestion.

Cardamom

It offers a unique aroma and flavor. There are many medical conditions you can relive using this Cardamom. Some of the common health problems you can cure at home include cholesterol control, relief from cardiovascular issues, control of cancer, and gastrointestinal protection.

Effectively taking one cardamom on the happening of acidity and even after every meal helps prevent the happening of the acidity. Crush one cardamom, then you need to put it in the water. Lastly, boil the water. The preparation is ready. Now you can consume the drink.

Basil

Basil is a great source of vitamin C, A, and iron, potassium, dietary fibers and calcium. It helps in indigestion. When experiencing a bloating problem, you can find a great cure with the help of basil. Chewing just a couple of leaves of it in the case of the prevalence of acidity is one high-quality natural medication for acidity as well as the discomfort the acidity brings.

Chapter 3. Acne

Aloe Vera

Aloe Vera, an herbal species is in use since the first century. Its leaves are used in the treatment for curing and softening the skin. You can use it for constipation as well as skin disorders. In fact, it can be used in different reasons. You can use it to relieve psoriasis, dandruff, seborrhea, skin abrasions, and minor burns. Recently, it has been shown that the aloe gel is very helpful in treating diabetes. It works by lowering the level of your blood sugar.

Comfortably apply the gel which comes out of the leaves for your face two times per day. Consume its juice every day with an empty belly in the morning. This will help reduce zits. You should have it in a pre-packaged as a substitute than pulling out the juice in uncooked kind. Making use of a combination of aloe Vera gel along with rosewater is as well a priceless home cure for acne.

Coriander

Coriander is rich in antioxidants, which causes your skin acne free. It also helps in detoxifying your skin, healing it from the happening of blackheads as well as acne. Coriander enables digestion, decreases fever, vomiting, as well as diarrhea. Coriander is usually beneficial in decreasing swelling or anguish. It contains various nutrients as well as minerals including iron, vitamin B1, B2, A, and C. Consumption of its water decreases the level of the cholesterol.

With the mixture of turmeric powder and coriander juice when utilized on the face you can benefit when experiencing blackheads and acne. It will have to be utilized after you wash your face at night. By using this juice on your face earlier than sleeping additionally helps can be an amazing home comfort for zits.

Chapter 4. Anxiety

Passion Flower-This is a typical sedative. It helps ease the happening of anxiety as well as stress.

Ginkgo Biloba –It is an herb that helps promote the temper by means of improving blood circulation.

Lemon Balm- It is soothing, as it helps get rid of restlessness brought about by means of anxiousness. When it comes to heart beat, this is something that can help. It helps cure nausea.

Ginseng-This herb is a stimulant as a result of it's a strong anti-depression property. It is a strong herbal remedy for anxiety, because it keeps emotional inequity.

California poppy-This natural sedative herb helps relieve stress as well as nervousness. It additionally eases the headache that can come up as a result of an anxiety attack.

Chamomile-It has more than a few advantages for various issues like sleep and belly problems. Chamomile tea can help reduce the event of anxiety attacks.

St. John's Wort-It is one kind of herb that is a common comfort for nervousness, as it's a strong anti depressant.

Kava-It is also an herb that is great for anxiety for rapid results. The outcomes of it can also be noticeable within a few weeks from the start of its use.

Chapter 5. Asthma

Figs

Figs had been particularly important within the average remedy for bronchial asthma. It is broadly used in the treatment of respiratory problems. This is a great home cure for asthma cough. It helps dry your phlegm.

To use figs, you need to use 4 figs. Then you should soak them in water. Let them stay overnight. You will drink the water in the morning.

Lemons

A lemon is considered an antibacterial and aid in getting rid of the germs the mucus has. In addition, they make faster restoration easy from a cough that leads to bronchial asthma attack. It additionally helps in cleansing the blood, making the lung tissues stronger.

Get a lemon. Extract its juice. Put it in one glass of water. Then, drink it with every meal. The combination regularly dissolves the bulky mucus within the bronchial tubes.

Safflower seeds

They are especially effective when it comes to bronchial asthma. Additionally, you will find help in treating the spasms. They are very beneficial. It is an effective remedy to decrease spasms. It works by making the mucus soft in the airways. 5 grams of those seeds with one tsp of organic honey can be a priceless remedy for bronchial asthma.

Chamomile

It works as a usual anesthetic to help decrease your stress via decreasing the outcomes of these chemical compounds which prompt stress. Chamomile helps in producing healthy adrenal hormones. It also helps in lessening the spasms. Chamomile tea will also be used two times a day for excellent results.

Chapter 6. Bloating

Turmeric

Turmeric has a range of nutrients including calcium, Vitamin C, protein, folic acid, and iron. It helps increase the digestive system's performance, easing bloating as well as gas. The digestion process makes easier, since it can help break down the proteins. It helps with bloating.

To successfully deal with bloating, this home relief can also be purchased in its powder type. Next, add it to a drink, or in your every meal. Take some times to experience the effect it offers. Include its powder to the meals or drink each time you think you bloat. Turmeric can also be found in tablet kind that can also be used orally to alleviate bloating.

Apple cider vinegar

This it helps in treating the bloating problem. To make it taste better, get some honey, and mix with it. This will make the vinegar sweeter. When experiencing bloating, take it a couple of minutes before your meals.

Mint leaves

Another natural relief for bloating is its leaves after you each meal. Get 3 leaves. Have leaves brewed along with the tea. Use the remedy twice a day to find a cure when experiencing a bloating problem.

Chapter 7. Bad Breath

Cloves

Making use of mouthwash or toothpaste containing clove will support to battle against dangerous breath. Additionally, using it in your ingredient will be the best healing for this problem.

Lemon

Lemon mouthwash is an efficient healing for your bad breath. Get one cup of warm water. Get half of one lemon. Mix into the water. Mix a bit of salt in the mixture. Gargle this mouthwash.

Celery

Celery is one of the most popular home remedies today. This is an herb most well-liked among that has too much cure efficiency. Its oil makes it fragrant in nature. It contains minerals, and nutrients. Celery is an effective home remedy to cure your bad breath. The reason it is highly effective to cure bad breath is that it has high fiber. Chewing celery can help increase the saliva production, keeping your mouth moist. Chewing it helps clean your tongue, a major source of bacteria that creates bad breath.

Peppermint

Add a plenty peppermint in a cup of water. Boil it. Eat this tea daily, two times a day to prevent your bad breath. Chew its leaves after every meal to freshen up your breath.

Chapter 8. Cough

Almonds

You need to first steep almonds in the water. After that get a paste ready after you eliminate their surface brown dermis. The paste must additionally comprise sugar as well as butter. Use it two times a day, in the morning and night hours. Soak as a minimum of 7 almonds in a single day, and prepare the paste.

Turmeric

This is another excellent herbal medicine that helps reduce your cough. The reason it is highly effective to cure your cough is that it contains curcuminoids. It works as an anti inflammatory agent. It has anti-bacterial as well as anti-viral action.

Cook and crush its root to give you a powder. Get the powder. You need to now get some carom powder to blend. Mix some water and make a paste. You would be able to mix some good quality honey. Take the combination thrice every day.

Black Pepper

One of the most effective remedies at home to help in managing your cough is Black Pepper. It is highly effective in removing mucus. It greatly helps open the chest clogging. Using it is very easy to reduce your cough. All of you need to do is take about 3 seeds of it, and chew.

Chapter 9. Common Cold

Lemon

One of the easiest natural home remedies to cure common cold is a lemon. It is rich in vitamin C that helps make the immune system stronger. Moreover, this vitamin C helps treat a variety of cold symptoms. Lemon has a major ability to reduce the growth of microbes. A microbe is something that causes infection. Eat 2 or 3 lemons a day when you are experiencing the common cold. It is better to eat it on a daily basis to prevent the possible problem. This is an effective way anyone can find the most benefits in treating common colds.

Garlic

In addition to many beneficial effects, garlic can help relieve your common cold problems. It contains antimicrobial as well as antiviral properties. They relieve the common cold effectively and naturally.

You can prepare garlic soup to reduce your colds. Take it every day. Get fresh cloves and bite them a couple of times per day. Get high-quality get garlic oil and blend it with onion in water, next drink this two times a day. Aside from relieving signs, you will be removing toxins from your body.

Ginger

Ginger has more than a few caring compounds such as allicin, the most powerful antibiotics. It has many anti-bacterial properties that boost the immunity to defeat the infection.

Boil the root in water. Stress and include sugar to drink the blend. Brewing ginger tea is another great method. Add the pieces of it in hot water and after that include tea leaves to make the drink extremely tasty. You can take two times a day to relieve your colds and coughs.

Coriander

Coriander has many health benefits. It has a cooling effect. It has been widely used in treating the most common cold. It can also help in the treatment of high cholesterol levels, inflammation, mouth ulcers, diarrhea, indigestion, anemia, smallpox, menstrual disorders, skin disorders, blood sugar disorders, and conjunctivitis.

Just crush it and leave to water. Cook this, and include sugar earlier than permitting it to calm. Heat it once more as long as you do not have a decoction that is wide and do away with from the fireplace. Take 4 times a day.

Chapter 10. Herpes

Cornstarch

Cornstarch is a fine powder used in the pharmaceutical industries. Using cornstarch and water you can easily create a paste. After that, keep using onto the field of illness. Then, this must be put down to dry as a technique of eliminating the itchiness.

Bitter melon

It will also help to soothe the sores. This is a simple home remedy for herpes. Use its extracts onto the infected area. This is an amazing way of eliminating herpes.

To use it for finding a relief from itching, you can get a cotton ball. Cold milk is something you should use when preparing the medication to treat your herpes. You need to dip the melon in the milk. Then use it to the affected part of your body.

Conclusion

Natural home remedies are merely ready treatment, or that contains substances produced from healthy solutions such as veggies fresh fruits along with spices or herbs. Additionally, it contains physical exercises, massaging, strategies, colors, fragrances, and detoxification. As a result of growing unwanted effects from the medications, consumers are today moving to different treatments for healing and also cure of typical medical problems. Home cures tend to be on the list of alternative techniques employed for treating typical illnesses in your own home.

With regard to home cures your kitchen is a wonderful place to begin. It offers just about all of your required medications to cope with popular conditions. Homemade remedies tend to be easy, affordable, without any negative effects, with no chemical substances. It needs 100 % natural ingredients, for example, fresh fruits, Veggies, natural herbs, in addition to Spices. Natural treatments work extremely well efficiently in treating a wide variety of conditions such as enhancing defense mechanisms, baldness, dealing with chronic acne breakouts, managing aches, burns, cuts, and much more.

Thank You Page

I want to personally thank you for reading my book. I hope you found information in this book useful and I would be very grateful if you could leave your honest review about this book. I certainly want to thank you in advance for doing this.

If you have the time, you can check my other books too.

www.ingramcontent.com/pod-product-compliance
Lightning Source LLC
Chambersburg PA
CBHW061935280526
45787CB00004B/1612

* 9 7 8 1 5 0 5 6 1 5 4 4 9 *